THE POWER OF 10:

10-Minute Workouts for Rapid Weight Loss

A Quick Fitness Guide for Busy People

BOBBY KINCAID

Legal Disclaimer:

The information provided in this book is for educational an

informational purposes only and is not intended to be a substitute fo

professional medical advice, diagnosis, or treatment. Always seek th

advice of your physician or other qualified healthcare providers with an

questions you may have regarding a medical condition or the suitabili

of any workout program. The author and publisher of this book are n

responsible for any adverse effects or consequences resulting from th

use of any suggestions, exercises, or information presented in this boo

The reader assumes full responsibility for any actions taken based on th

information in this book.

Table of Contents

I

Introduction

ey there, my fellow busy 9 to 5-er! Are you tired of reminiscing about
e "good old days" when you had all the time and energy in the world to
ork out? Better yet, maybe you didn't need a workout plan because you
e whatever you wanted, whenever you wanted, and never gained a
und. Do you find yourself scrolling through your old high school
otos, wishing you could magically transport yourself back to your
enage physique? Trust me; I've been there. But here's the thing: you
n't need a time machine to get back in shape.

et me introduce myself. I'm Bobby, and like many of you, I was in great
ape during my high school days. I had plenty of energy, a faster
etabolism, and free time to spare. But then came the 9-5 grind. I spent
ost of my days sitting in front of a computer, and by the time I got
me, I was too tired to even think about working out. Sound familiar?

r a while, I tried to force myself to hit the gym for an hour or more
ery day. But between work, errands, and social commitments, it just
asn't sustainable. I began to feel discouraged and wondered if I'd ever
 able to get back to my old self.

ut then, I discovered the power of 10-minute workouts. At first, I was
eptical. 10 minutes? That's barely enough time to warm up, right? But

as I started experimenting with shorter workouts, I realized I was getting as much (if not more) out of them as I did from longer sessions.

Not only did these short workouts help me to maintain my physique, but they also had a positive impact on my overall health and well-being. I had more energy throughout the day, slept better at night, and felt more confident in my own skin.

And the best part? I didn't have to sacrifice my entire evening to do it. With 10-minute workouts, I could get a solid sweat in before heading to work in the morning or during a lunch break and still have plenty of time for other activities and socializing.

In this book, I will show you how to get the most out of your 10-minute workouts. We'll cover everything from quick and effective exercises to tips for staying motivated and avoiding burnout. And don't worry; I'm not going to bore you with complicated fitness jargon or impossible-to-follow routines. I will break down everything into simple, easy-to-follow steps that even your teenage self could understand.

So if you're ready to ditch the desk and get back to your teenage physique (well, as close as possible, at least), let's do this. We'll laugh, we'll sweat, and who knows? Maybe we'll even make a few new high school-esque memories along the way. It's time to make 10 minutes count!

Why 10-Minute Workouts Are a Game Changer

Why spend hours at the gym without seeing any real results?

Why start a rigorous workout routine and not have time or energy to be consistent?

Most of us have busy lives and can't afford to spend hours on end exercising. You don't need to be a superhero or a supermodel to achieve your fitness goals. **All you need is the power of 10!**

Now, I know what you're thinking - how can such a short workout be effective? Well, the answer lies in the science behind it. Studies have shown that short, high-intensity workouts can be just as effective if not more effective, than longer, low-intensity workouts.

When you perform high-intensity exercises, you activate your body's anaerobic energy systems, which help you burn fat and build muscle. Research has shown that a 10-minute high-intensity workout can burn as many calories as a 30-minute jog!

But enough with the scientific facts (for now). Let's get back to the fun stuff. Remember those movie-action heroes we all love and admire? Think about their training routines - they rarely spend hours upon hours in the gym, but instead, they focus on short, intense workouts to build strength, endurance, and agility. They know that time is precious, and they use it wisely.

And for all the ladies out there, let's not forget about the runway supermodels. They have tight schedules, jet lag, and busy lives, just like you. But they stay in shape by incorporating short, high-intensity workouts into their daily routines. They know that a quick sweat session can boost their metabolism and give them the extra energy they need to conquer the day. You don't have to be an Instagram "fitness guru/ influencer" to be ready for hot girl summer.

All you need is the power of 10!

So, what are the true benefits of short, high-intensity workouts, you may ask? Well, there are many! In the next section, we'll dive into the specifics, but here's a quick rundown:

- They're time-efficient
- They boost your metabolism
- They help you burn fat and build muscle
- They improve your cardiovascular health
- They increase your energy levels

The list goes on, but you get the idea. So, let's put those 10 minutes to good use and get started on the journey to a stronger, healthier, and happier you!

The True Benefits of short workouts

Ok, hold on to your wigs & caps! We're going to get a bit technical, but don't worry; we'll break it down for you in a way even Tony Stark's AI system, Jarvis, can appreciate it. And for those of you who prefer the brute strength of the Incredible Hulk & SheHulk, we'll be sure to include some muscle-building tips as well. So, without further ado, let's explore the true benefits of short workouts.

#1 Time Efficiency

Let's face it, we all have busy lives. Between work, family, and other obligations, finding time to exercise can be a challenge. But with short workouts, you can achieve maximum results in minimal time—no more excuses about not having enough time to hit the gym or go for a run. With just 10 minutes a day, you can get in a full-body workout that will leave you feeling energized and accomplished.

#2 Boosts Metabolism

Short, high-intensity workouts boost metabolism, allowing your body to burn more calories throughout the day. This means you can burn fat while sitting at your desk or even while sleeping! It's like having your fat burning furnace that never shuts off.

#3 Burns Fat and Builds Muscle

Short workouts are also great for building lean muscle mass and burning fat. By incorporating exercises that target multiple muscle groups, you can achieve a full-body workout that will help you shed unwanted pounds and tone your body.

#4 Improves Cardiovascular Health

Cardiovascular exercise is essential for maintaining a healthy heart and reducing your risk of heart disease. Short workouts incorporating high intensity interval training (HIIT) improve cardiovascular health and increase endurance; more on that later.

#5 Increases Energy Levels

It may seem counterintuitive, but short workouts can increase your energy levels. Regular exercise boosts energy and reduces fatigue, and quick workouts are no exception. By getting your blood pumping and leasing endorphins, you'll feel energized and ready to take on whatever e day throws your way.

the next chapter, we'll go deeper into the science of short workouts and ow you how to incorporate them into your busy lifestyle. So grab a otein shake, and let's get started!

II

The Science of Short Workouts

Welcome to the nitty-gritty, a brief deep dive into the science behind short workouts and why they're so effective. Don't worry; we'll get back to all the fun in due course.

First, let's talk about how to maximize results with shorter workouts. Short workouts are about intensity, so you must make every minute count. Be sure you are doing exercises that work multiple muscle groups simultaneously, like squats, push-ups, and lunges. You can also use equipment like kettlebells or resistance bands to up the intensity.

Another way to maximize results is to incorporate high-intensity interval training (HIIT) into your workouts. HIIT involves short bursts of intense exercise followed by periods of rest or lower-intensity exercise. One significant benefit is that it helps you burn fat and build muscle simultaneously. By pushing yourself to your limits during those short bursts of high-intensity exercise, you're stimulating muscle growth and improving your body's ability to burn fat. This means you'll see results faster than with traditional steady-state cardio. When you do short, intense exercises, you activate a process called EPOC (Excess Post-Exercise Oxygen Consumption), which keeps your body burning calories even after your workout is over. What many like to call "after burn," and YES! in a good way.

Another benefit of HIIT is that it improves your cardiovascular health. HIIT workouts get your heart rate up and challenge your heart and lungs, which can improve your overall cardiovascular fitness. Plus, it can help lower your blood pressure and reduce your risk of heart disease.

Now, let's get into some examples of HIIT exercises. One of my favorites is the Tabata protocol. This protocol is a type of HIIT that involves short bursts of intense exercise followed by even shorter rest periods. The whole workout usually lasts about 4 minutes, but don't be fooled by the short duration - it can be a challenging workout!

The basic idea is to perform an exercise at maximum effort for 20 seconds, then rest for 10 seconds. You repeat this 20 seconds on, 10 seconds off pattern for a total of 8 cycles or rounds, which comes out to 4 minutes in total.

The Tabata Protocol is great for busy people like you who don't have much time to exercise but still want to get a good workout. And the best part is that it's super versatile - you can do Tabata with almost any exercise, from bodyweight moves like squats and push-ups to cardio exercises like burpees or jump rope.

Another example is the EMOM (every minute on the minute) protocol. EMOM is a workout protocol where you perform a specific exercise or set of exercises at the top of every minute for a predetermined amount of time.

For example, if you were doing an EMOM workout of 10 minutes with push-ups, you would do a set of push-ups at the start of every minute, resting for the remaining time until the next minute starts. The key to the EMOM protocol is to complete each set of exercises within the minute so you have time to rest before the next set. The idea is to keep your heart rate elevated while allowing enough recovery time to push through the entire workout.

EMOM workouts can be a great way to challenge yourself and build endurance. Plus, they're customizable to fit any fitness level or goal. You can adjust the number of exercises, the workout duration, and the intensity of each exercise to make it work for you.

So there you have it, that wasn't so bad. You now know the science behind short workouts and how to maximize your results with HIIT. Incorporating these principles into your workout routine can help you achieve your fitness goals quickly. In the next chapter, we'll move into designing effective 10-minute workouts that work for your individual needs and goals.

III

Designing Effective 10-Minute Workouts

lright, If you've been following along, you now know the benefits of orter workouts and the science behind them. But how do you design a lanced 10-minute workout that's effective?

emember, it's crucial to ensure that your workout hits all the major uscle groups. This means including exercises for your chest, back, legs, ms, and core. And no, doing endless bicep curls won't cut it.

'hen designing your workout, think about compound exercises. For ample, squats work not only your legs but also your core and glutes. ush-ups work your chest, triceps, and shoulders while engaging your re.

addition to compound exercises, it's also essential to include some rm of cardiovascular exercise in your 10-minute workout. This can be simple as jumping jacks, mountain climbers, or burpees. Not only will is help increase your heart rate, but it'll also help you burn more calories a shorter amount of time.

ow, let's talk about some key exercises to include in your 10-minute orkout. We've already mentioned squats and push-ups, but other great exercises include lunges, planks, rows, and shoulder presses. These exercises effectively target multiple muscle groups and can easily be modified to fit your fitness level.

Speaking of fitness levels, let's examine some sample 10-minute workouts for different fitness levels. Remember, these are just examples you can always modify them to fit your needs.

For beginners, a sample 10-minute workout might look something like this:

- 30 seconds of jumping jacks
- 10 squats
- 10 push-ups (Modified: on your knees if needed)
- 10 lunges (5 on each leg)
- 30-second plank
- 10 mountain climbers
- 10-second rest

For intermediate fitness levels, you might try this 10-minute workout:

- 30 seconds of high knees
- 15 squats
- 15 push-ups
- 15 rows (using resistance bands or dumbbells)
- 30-second plank with shoulder taps
- 15 burpees
- 15-second rest

And for those who are more advanced, try this 10-minute workout:

- 30 seconds of jump squats
- 20 push-ups
- 20 lunges (10 on each leg)
- 20 rows (using resistance bands or dumbbells)
- 30-second plank with hip dips
- 20 burpees
- 10-second rest

Remember, these are just example sets, and you can always modify the exercises or the time intervals to fit your fitness level and preference. With some creativity and critical exercises, you can design an effective 10-minute workout that fits even the busiest of schedules.

Step-By-Step Guides

While some of these exercises may appear simple, it's vital to ensure proper form to prevent potential injuries. For those unfamiliar with these exercises, here are step-by-step instructions on how to perform them correctly.

Jumping Jacks

Here's a step-by-step guide to performing jumping jacks with proper form:

1. Start with your feet together and your arms at your sides.
2. Next, jump up, spreading your feet shoulder-width apart as you do so.
3. As you jump, raise your arms above your head to form a "V" shape.
4. Jump back to the starting position, bringing your feet back together and lowering your arms to your sides.
5. Repeat steps 2-4 for the desired number of repetitions.

It's crucial to maintain good posture throughout the exercise. Keep your chest up and your shoulders back, and engage your core to help stabilize your body.

Also, be sure to land softly on the balls of your feet rather than your heels to reduce the impact on your joints. This can help prevent injury and make the exercise more comfortable.

Finally, be sure to breathe normally throughout the exercise. Inhale as you jump up, and exhale as you jump back down.

By following these steps and maintaining proper form, you can get the most out of your jumping jacks and avoid injury.

Squats

Here's a step-by-step guide to performing squats with proper form:

1. Start with your feet shoulder-width apart, toes pointing forward or slightly outwards.
2. Engage your core and keep your chest up, shoulders back, and spine neutral.
3. Lower your body by bending at the knees and pushing your hips back as if sitting on a chair. Keep your weight on your heels and your knees tracking over your toes.
4. Lower your body until your thighs are parallel to the floor or slightly below while maintaining good form.
5. Drive through your heels and stand back up, squeezing your glutes at the top.
6. Repeat for the desired number of repetitions.

It's essential to avoid common mistakes like rounding your lower back, letting your knees cave in, or allowing your heels to come off the ground. By keeping good form and engaging the right muscles, you can get the most out of your squats and avoid unnecessary injuries.

Planks

Here's a step-by-step guide to performing planks with proper form:

1. Begin by placing your forearms on the ground, shoulder-width apart, with your elbows directly under your shoulders.
2. Extend your legs straight behind you, with your toes on the ground and your feet hip-width apart.
3. Engage your core muscles by drawing your navel towards your spine and squeezing your glutes to help stabilize your body.
4. Keep your neck neutral by looking at the ground about a foot in front of you.
5. Hold this position for the desired time, maintaining proper form throughout.
6. To avoid injury, make sure not to let your lower back sag or raise your hips too high. Also, keep your body in a straight line from head to heels.
7. When you're ready to finish the exercise, slowly lower yourself to the ground by coming down onto your knees, then onto your stomach.

Remember to start with shorter holds and gradually increase your time as your core strength improves. By maintaining proper form, you'll maximize the benefits of the exercise while minimizing the risk of injury.

Planks with Shoulder Taps

Here is a step-by-step guide to performing planks with shoulder taps with proper form:

1. Begin by getting into a high plank position with your hands shoulder-width apart on the ground and your feet hip-width apart. Keep your body in a straight line from your head to your heels.
2. Engage your core muscles and glutes by pulling your belly button inward towards your spine and squeezing your buttocks.
3. Keeping your hips as stable as possible, lift your right hand off the ground and tap your left shoulder.
4. Return your right hand to the ground and repeat on the other side, lifting your left hand off the ground and tapping your right shoulder.
5. Continue alternating shoulder taps for the desired amount of time or repetitions.

Important form tips to keep in mind:

- Keep your elbows straight and your shoulders directly over your wrists throughout the exercise.
- Keep your head and neck neutral, looking down towards the ground.
- Focus on maintaining a stable core and avoiding any twisting or rotation in your hips.
- Keep your feet hip-width apart or slightly wider for greater stability.

Push-ups

ere are the steps to properly perform a push-up with good form:

1. Start in a high plank position with your hands slightly wider than shoulder-width apart, fingers facing forward, and your body in a straight line from head to heels.
2. Lower your body down towards the ground, keeping your elbows close to your body until your chest almost touches the ground.
3. Pause briefly when your chest is close to the ground.
4. Push your body back up to the starting position by extending your arms fully.
5. Repeat the movement, keeping your body straight and rigid throughout the exercise.

ome tips for maintaining good form:

- Keep your elbows close to your body throughout the movement.
- Avoid letting your hips sag or sticking your butt up in the air. Instead, your body should remain straight from head to heels.
- Focus on engaging your chest, triceps, and shoulders to lift your body rather than using your lower back or hips to cheat the movement.
- Breathe in as you lower your body towards the ground and exhale as you push back up to the starting position.

s essential to start with the proper form, even if that means doing fewer reps modifying the exercise. Then, gradually increase the number of reps and ts as you get stronger and more comfortable with the movement.

Lunges

Here's a step-by-step guide to performing lunges with proper form:

1. Stand with your feet hip-width apart and your hands on your hips or by your sides.
2. Take a big step forward with one leg, keeping your torso upright.
3. Lower your body until your front thigh is parallel to the ground and your back knee is hovering just above the ground. Both your front and back legs should form 90-degree angles.
4. Ensure your front knee stays above your ankle and does not extend past your toes.
5. Push through your front heel to return to the starting position.
6. Repeat with the opposite leg.

Some additional tips to keep in mind when performing lunges:

- Keep your core engaged in helping maintain your balance.
- Don't let your front knee cave inward - keep it in line with your toe
- Keep your back straight, and your shoulders relaxed.
- Take slow and controlled steps to avoid losing balance.

By following these steps and tips, you can perform lunges with prop form and reduce the risk of injury.

Rows (with resistance bands or dumbbells)

Here's a step-by-step guide to performing rows with proper form:

1. Stand with your feet shoulder-width apart and hold the resistance band or dumbbells with an overhand grip. Extend your arms in front of you, and your palms should face downward.
2. Brace your core and keep your spine straight, with your shoulders pulled back and down.
3. Begin the rowing motion by pulling the resistance band or dumbbells towards your body, with your elbows close to your sides. Imagine that you are pulling your shoulder blades toward each other.
4. Keep your wrists straight and your forearms perpendicular to the ground.
5. Pause for a moment when you reach the top of the movement, making sure to squeeze your shoulder blades together.
6. Slowly release the resistance band or dumbbells back to the starting position with control. Do not allow the weight to pull you back into a slouched position.

Remember to keep your movements controlled and smooth throughout the exercise. Avoid jerking or swinging your arms to generate momentum. This can cause injury and decrease the effectiveness of the exercise.

If using a resistance band, make sure to secure it to an anchor point or use a door attachment to avoid it slipping during the exercise.

Burpees

Here's a step-by-step guide to performing burpees with proper form:

1. Start in a standing position with your feet shoulder-width apart.
2. Drop down into a squat position with your hands on the floor in front of you.
3. Kick your feet back so that you're in a push-up position with your arms extended.
4. Lower your body to the ground, keeping your elbows close to your body.
5. Push yourself back up into a push-up position.
6. Jump your feet back up to the squat position.
7. Stand up straight, jump into the air, and clap your hands above your head.

Some additional tips to keep in mind:

- Keep your core tight and engaged throughout the movement to protect your lower back.
- Ensure your chest touches the ground when you lower your body into the push-up position.
- Land softly when you jump back up to the squat position to avoid any jarring impact on your joints.
- As you jump into the air, try to get as much height as possible to engage your leg muscles more effectively.

By following these tips and maintaining proper form, you can get the most out of your burpee workouts while minimizing the risk of injury.

IV

How to Maximize Your Results

udos on making it this far! You've learned about the benefits of short
orkouts and how to design an effective 10-minute routine. Now, let's
lk about how to make the most of those 10 minutes.

ne of the keys to maximizing your results is to push yourself during
ur workout. Remember, you only have a limited amount of time, so
u need to make every second count. This doesn't mean that you should
crifice proper form, but it does mean that you should challenge yourself
ith each exercise.

ere are some tips to help you push yourself during your 10-minute
orkout:

- Set a goal: Before you start your workout, set a specific goal for
  what you want to achieve. Write it down and track your progress!
  Maybe you want to do 10 push-ups without stopping or hold a plank
  for 30 seconds longer than last time. Having a goal in mind can help
  you stay focused and motivated.
- Use the correct weight: If you're using weights, ensure you use the
  right weight for your fitness level. You should be able to complete

each set with proper form, but the last few reps should be challenging.

- Incorporate high-intensity intervals: High-intensity intervals, like the ones discussed, can help you burn more calories and improve your fitness level over time.

While pushing yourself during your workout is essential, it's also important to avoid common mistakes that can lead to injury or prevent you from getting the most out of your training.

Here are some common mistakes to avoid:

- Sacrificing form for speed: While challenging yourself is important, it's never okay to sacrifice proper form. Doing an exercise with improper form not only increases your risk of injury but can also reduce the effectiveness of the exercise.
- Neglecting rest days: Rest days are just as important as workout days. Your body needs time to recover and repair itself, so make sure you're incorporating rest days into your fitness routine. Pick 1-2 days in between your weekly routine to rest.
- Not listening to your body: It's essential to push yourself, but it's also important to listen to your body. If something doesn't feel right

stop and take a break. Pushing through pain or discomfort can lead to injury.

Lastly, staying motivated can be challenging, especially when you're short on time. Here are some tips to help you stay motivated during your 10-minute workouts:

- Set a routine: Try to stick to a consistent workout routine. This can help you develop a habit and make it easier to stay motivated. (i.e., M, W, F, Sat)
- Find a workout buddy: Working out with a friend or family member can be a great way to stay motivated and accountable.
- Celebrate your progress: Take time to celebrate your progress, no matter how small it may seem. Celebrating your progress can help you stay motivated and inspired to keep going.

Remember, making the most of your 10-minute workout is about pushing yourself, avoiding common mistakes, and staying motivated. With these tips, you can achieve your fitness goals and maximize your limited time.

V

Incorporating 10-Minute Workouts into Your Busy Life

Ah, the eternal struggle to find time for exercise amidst our busy lives. Fear not, for I have some ideas to help you incorporate 10-minute workouts into your daily routine.

First off, let's address the elephant in the room: time. We all have the same 24 hours in a day, but it's how we use them that matters. So, let's get creative. You can break up your 10-minute workouts throughout the day, doing a few exercises in the morning, a few during your lunch break, and a few before bed. You can also try waking up 10 minutes earlier to get your sweat on.

If you find yourself constantly on the go, there are still ways to fit in short workouts. Try doing some exercises while waiting in line or on a phone call. I mean, what better way to catapult yourself to the front of the Chipotle line while others make room for the crazy person who spontaneously bursts into an array of jumping jacks? No really, there's no excuse for why you can't find the time. You could even do some simple stretches or squats during commercial breaks while watching TV. These might be bizarre mentions, but hey, whatever it takes to get the job done.

Also, if you're like me and tend to procrastinate, schedule your 10-minute workout into your day. Treat it like any other appointment that you can't miss. After all, exercise is just as important as that meeting with your boss or that lunch date with your bestie.

Lastly, consistency is key. It's important to make exercise a part of your daily routine, even if it's just 10 minutes a day. It's not about going hard for one day and then giving up altogether. It's about making small changes that add up over time. So, don't beat yourself up if you miss a day; get back on track the next day.

Incorporating 10-minute workouts into your life may take effort and creativity, but it's worth it. With a little determination and a positive mindset, you can easily make exercise a regular part of your daily routine.

VI

Hydration, Nutrition, and Recovery

People often overlook hydration, nutrition, and recovery, but they are just as important as the workout itself. Let's talk about how to hydrate & fuel your body for those short but intense workouts and how to recover properly to maximize your results.

Hydration

Did you know that our bodies are mostly made up of water? It's on Google, so it must be true! In fact, on average, about 60% of our body weight is made up of water. That means if you weigh 150 pounds, about 90 of those pounds are water. Crazy, right?

Water is crucial for our bodies to function correctly. It helps regulate our body temperature, carries nutrients to our cells, and aids digestion. Hydration is key! It's essential to drink water before, during, and after your workout. Your body needs water to function correctly and to replenish the fluids lost during exercise. So, grab your water bottle and take a sip before we continue.

Try an IV…

Liquid IV, that is. It's a fantastic product that can give your workouts a boost! It works by providing your body with the hydration it needs to keep you performing at your best. When you sweat, your body loses vital fluids and electrolytes, making you feel exhausted and crampy. Liquid IV replenishes these essential nutrients and helps you maintain optimal hydration levels. This can lead to better performance, endurance, and faster recovery times.

But that's not all - Liquid IV also contains essential vitamins and minerals that support overall health and wellness. For example, vitamin C and potassium help boost your immune system and reduce inflammation, while B vitamins boost natural energy. This means you can power through your workouts and feel great doing them!

This is not a sponsored ad, but if we were on social media, by this point, I'd be asking you to subscribe now, punch that like button and tag me in your feed. Yet we're not; either way, if you feel you've gotten some value out of what you read so far, I guess I'll have to settle for a glowing review. appreciate any help you can provide.

Nutrition

Now back to it, let's talk about fueling your body. Eating a balanced diet s essential for any fitness regimen. Make sure to consume carbohydrates, protein, and healthy fats to give your body the energy it needs. Complex carbohydrates like whole grains and vegetables will provide sustained energy throughout your workout, while protein will help repair and build muscle. Don't forget about healthy fats, like those found in nuts and avocados, as they also play a role in providing energy and aiding in recovery.

f you want to get the most out of your workouts, you need to pay ttention to what you eat and when you eat it. You'll want to fuel up with a meal high in carbs and protein. Aim to eat about 2-3 hours before your workout to give your body enough time to digest. But if you're short on ime, no worries! Grab a piece of fruit or a protein bar about 30 minutes before you start sweating.

After you crush your workout, it's crucial to give your muscles the utrition they need to recover. Load up again on foods high in protein and arbs, like chicken and rice or a hearty salad with quinoa. And if you're ooking for something quick and easy, a protein shake or smoothie is a great option too. Just ensure you're giving your body what it needs to repair and rebuild those muscles.

Recovery

Now, let's talk about recovery. Rest is just as important as exercise when it comes to seeing results. Make sure to give your body enough time to rest and recover between workouts. This means getting enough sleep, stretching, and foam rolling to aid muscle recovery. Incorporating proper nutrition and recovery strategies into your fitness routine can help you see better results and prevent injury.

I cannot stress the importance of hydration, nutrition, and recovery in achieving your fitness goals enough. It may sound cliché, but, indeed you cannot out-exercise a bad diet. It's crucial to break the habit of neglecting proper nutrition and not allowing your body to rest and recover adequately. Remember that taking care of your body and giving it what it needs will not only help you reach your fitness goals but also lead to better overall health and well-being. So make sure to prioritize hydration, nutrition, and recovery in your fitness journey, and watch as your progress skyrockets!

VII

Beyond 10 Minutes: Building on Your Progress

Great job on completing 10-minute workouts! You've built a solid foundation of fitness that you can now use to push yourself even further. In this chapter, we'll discuss how to progress your workouts beyond 10 minutes, incorporate longer workouts into your routine, and set achievable fitness goals.

Firstly, when it comes to progressing your workouts beyond 10 minutes, there are a few things you can do. One option is to increase the intensity of your workouts by adding more weight, increasing the reps or sets, or decreasing your rest time between exercises. This will challenge your body to adapt to new stress levels, leading to greater strength and endurance gains.

Another option is to try new exercises or variations of exercises you already know. Include an uptempo 10-minute walk on the treadmill with a high incline. This keeps your body guessing and helps prevent plateaus. You can also incorporate more complex movements, such as plyometrics or Olympic lifts, to challenge your coordination and athleticism.

When it comes to incorporating longer workouts into your routine, it's essential to increase your training volume to avoid overtraining or injury gradually. This can be done by adding an extra workout day to your week, gradually increasing the duration of your workouts, or doing a combination of both.

It's also important to vary the types of workouts you do. For example, you might alternate between strength training and cardiovascular exercise or try a new activity like pilates or aerobics. This will help prevent boredom and ensure that you are challenging your body in different ways.

Finally, setting and achieving fitness goals is vital to staying motivated and progressing. Start by selecting a specific, measurable goal, such as running a 5K or doing 10 pull-ups. Break this larger goal into smaller, achievable steps and create a plan to work towards them. Celebrate each small victory along the way and keep pushing yourself to reach new heights. I mean, even if you set out to look good in your birthday suit, go for it and let it all hang out. Heck! Find a local boudoir photographer and go for it; treat yourself for all that hard work you put into getting the results you desire. Make it a personal keepsake for you and your present or future spouse, and revisit it every other year.

Remember, fitness is a journey, not a destination. By continuing to challenge yourself and stay committed to your goals, you can build a healthier, stronger, and more resilient body. So go ahead and keep pushing beyond 10 minutes - your body will thank you!

VIII

Conclusion

ongratulations, you made it to the end of this book! You're now
quipped with the knowledge and tools to make 10-minute workouts a
ime-changer in your fitness journey. Let's quickly recap some key
oints we've covered throughout this book.

'e began by discussing the true benefits of short workouts, including
aving time, increasing consistency and high intensity, improving
rdiovascular health, building strength and endurance, boosting
etabolism and weight loss, reducing stress, and finally, improving
ental health. These benefits are backed by the science, which shows that
en just 10 minutes of exercise can have significant health benefits. We
aximize our results by incorporating short workouts into our busy lives,
d by consistently doing so we can achieve our fitness goals and live
ealthier.

ext, we explored how to incorporate these workouts into your busy life,
hether it's through quick and convenient exercises you can do at home
finding opportunities to move throughout the day. We delve into the
iportance of hydration, nutrition and recovery for short workouts,

including the best ways to fuel your body before and after exercise and strategies for augmented results.

Remember, progress takes time and consistency, but the most important thing is to keep going. Don't let setbacks discourage you - use them as opportunities to learn and grow. You got this!

Take advantage of the power of 10 and start incorporating 10-minute workouts into your life. Have fun, be creative, and most importantly enjoy the journey!

Made in the USA
Monee, IL
28 April 2023

32636308R00030